APPLE CIDER VINEGAR?

LET ME EXPLAIN

I0419573

"Everything you need to know... and more"

Pearl Robinson

DISCLAIMER

This book is not intended as a substitute for the medical advice of physicians. The reader should regularly consult a physician in matters relating to his/her health and particularly with respect to any symptoms that may require diagnosis or medical attention.

Table of Contents

Contents

Introduction

You are reading this book to learn more about one of the most intriguing, effective and affordable health tonics known to humanity. You would have heard – perhaps vaguely – about the potency of Apple Cider Vinegar (ACV), but were not convinced because you did not have any real data, facts or explanations.

This book will introduce you to ACV as it is popularly known, and as you learn about its amazing properties and powers, you will learn to love it and revere it as one of the most remarkable gifts of Mother Nature.

The best part of Apple Cider Vinegar is that it is most affordable. It is a simple recipe that you could make at home at negligible cost. Yet, the health benefits that you can enjoy from this humble compound are mind-boggling. To give a quick idea, ACV is often dubbed as the "Fountain of Youth" or "Elixir of Life".

Additionally, it doubles as a natural, non-toxic cleaner and a highly effective pest repellant. As you read through pages of this book, you will be amazed at the versatility this ONE compound offers. It is like a miracle potion that offers you unending boons.

This is one thing that every human being, every family should know about and use. It can change your life to a large extent, making you healthy, more energetic, more mentally alert, and more youthful looking. If that is not enough, it also increases longevity. There are people who swear by its veracity; people who have lived productive and active lives of up to 120 years.

Though everything that is presented in this Book is tried and tested, it is STRONGLY recommended that you do not take up anything that can affect your health without first consulting a doctor. This is very important.

Thank you for downloading and reading this Book. I hope you will have fun and benefit plenty from it. At the end of the Book, there are some useful and free (aren't the best things free?) resources that will provide more insights and interesting information about ACV.

Have fun!

Chapter 1: Apple Cider Vinegar (ACV) – What Is This?

A Little Background History

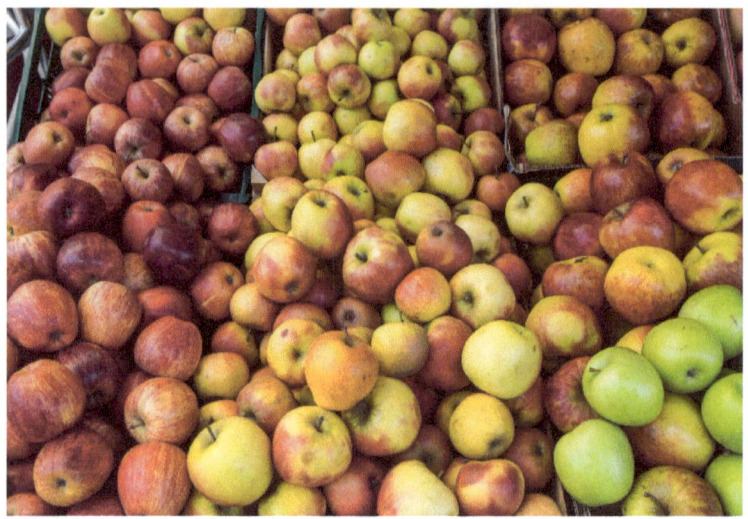

Apple Cider Vinegar or ACV as it is popularly known all over the world, is simply vinegar made from apples. This vinegar is a rich source of acetic acid as all vinegars are; additionally, it is a wealth of nutrients that provide virtually an unlimited list of benefits. People who are ACV fans will swear by it as a handy solution for innumerable health conditions with an added bonus, i.e. it is an amazing cleaning agent, as well.

Using Apple Cider Vinegar as a health remedy goes back to the time when ancient civilizations of Egypt, Greece, Babylon, and the Roman Empire thrived. Historical records show that the Father of Medicine, Hippocrates himself was treating patients with ACV and honey in circa 400 BC.

In ancient Egypt – about 3,000 BCE – the vinegar was used to cure many ailments; there is enough historic proof to back this up. The

Roman Empire during Julius Caesar's reign used ACV as a tonic for its army for energy and to fight infection. It is said that Christopher Columbus always stocked his ships with barrels of ACV before launching for any expedition as this helped keep his sailors free from scurvy – a deadly disease from Vitamin C deficiency.

In Europe, it was used as "youth elixir" and an extremely potent deodorant. Its legendary properties to fight infection and maintain a youthful skin made it a must-have ingredient in every woman's health and beauty home-remedy kit.

As Dr. Simon Yu, MD puts it, this simple ingredient offers humanity benefits that no other compound does. The amazing thing is that ACV is within the reach of anyone who want to use it hence, it has no limitations as other exotic health tonics/ remedies do. Anyone can use it. So, why aren't you? Perhaps because you are not yet convinced about the powerhouse of goodness it is.

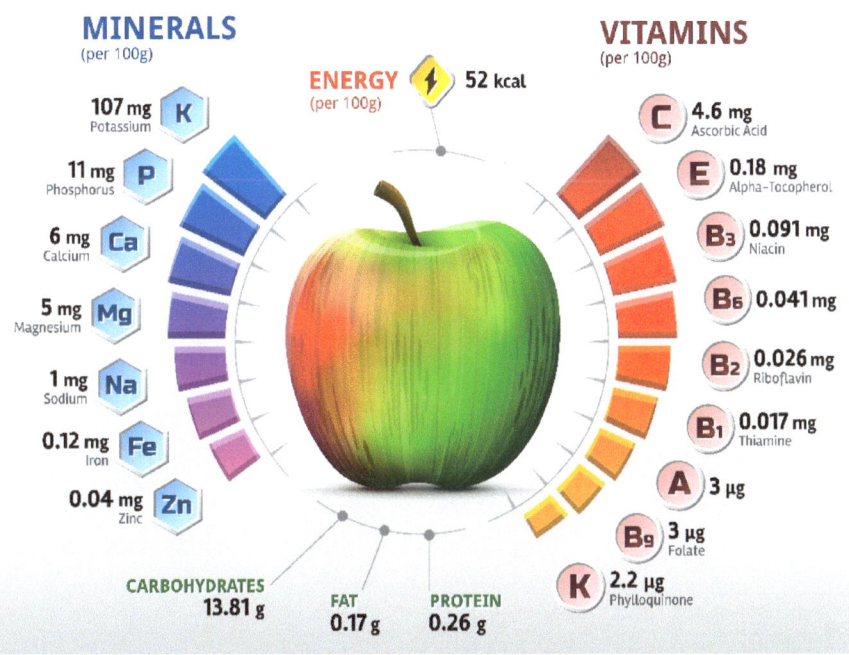

Take a quick look at the benefits this amazing ingredient offers you. Most of these benefits will be described in greater detail in the following chapters.

- Alkalizes your body, hence, making it disease resistant
- Protects your heart
- Detoxifies your body
- Aids digestions
- Improves nutrients assimilation
- Balances the pH in the body
- Kills germs
- Kills viruses
- Kills bacteria
- Kills fungus
- Helps with weight loss as it attacks the fat in the body
- Reverses ageing symptoms on skin
- Counters skin dryness
- Prevents hair loss and gives the hair gloss and body
- Enhances energy levels
- Rich source of vital minerals such as potassium, iron, boron and trace elements
- Rich source of enzymes and organic acids

...and this is only the tip of the iceberg.

Prevention And Healing – http://www.preventionandhealing.com – Simon Yu, MD, Board Certified Internist, who practices medicine with focus on Alternative Medicine.

To enjoy the benefits of ACV, you need to choose the right one. Either make it at home (check out the recipes given in this book) or buy from reputed brands

The raw organic vinegar is the one to look for; NOT the distilled one, because the distilled one is dead. The raw organic one is alive with nutrients, enzymes, minerals which interact with your body's systems to provide a basketful of health benefits. You will know that the vinegar is "alive" if it has a deposit at the bottom. This deposit is known as "mother". If there is no deposit, the vinegar is distilled and hence, dead; this is okay for taste, but will offer no health benefit. The vinegar with *"mother"* is the one you should look for. The natural, raw vinegar is orange-brown in color, has a pungent odor and a very visible *"mother"*.

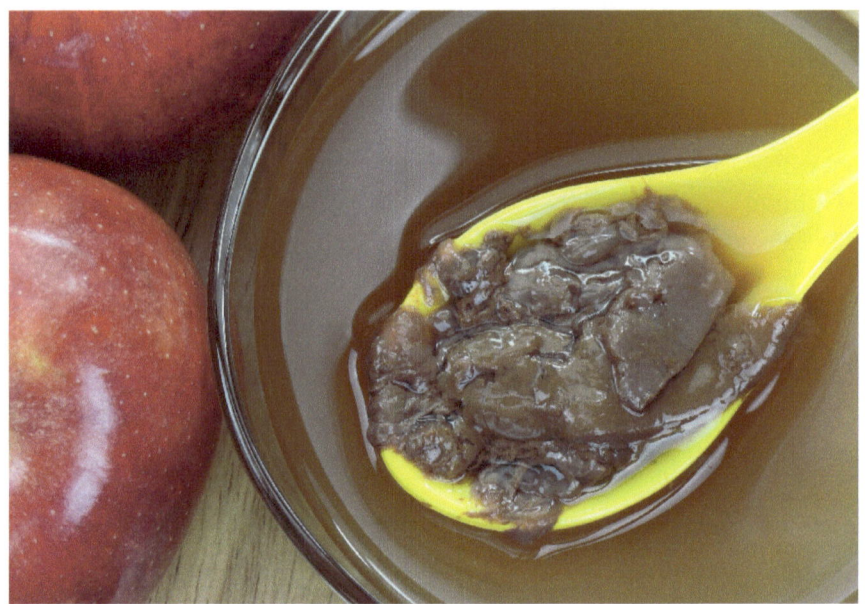

Unfortunately, to the uninformed, the natural, full-of-benefits ACV does not look as good as its distilled, clear and sparkling distilled counterpart. People tend to choose the "pretty" vinegar rather than the "ugly" vinegar with the visible "mother". This is perhaps the reason why the ACV – once a common product in all grocery stores – has almost disappeared from the market.

How to Buy ACV?

You can buy ACV online or from specific grocery shops. It may sound like a no-brainer, but there are a few things that you should be aware of before you make a purchase. There are TWO types, one is the organic, unpasteurized and "alive" one and the other type is "dead" or distilled. For maximum health benefits, you need to purchase the organic ACV, which is alive. Here are the aspects you should look for:

- It is a pale amber color or light brown.

- When you buy ACV, ensure that the label mentions "mother enzyme". The mother enzyme looks something like a spider's web floating in the liquid, which to the uninformed looks like it is spoilt. It is not. The label should read "organic" and mention "mother enzyme".

- Buy it raw. This means that the ACV is not treated, it has not been filtered and no artificial flavors have been offered to make it tastier, sweeter, or better flavored. In other words, you need your ACV unheated, unpasteurized, unprocessed and unfiltered.

- Stay away from the "sparkling" ones. When it is about ACV, the ugliest are the best.

- Buy ONLY the ACV bottled in glass bottles. No matter what the claims are, the plastic bottles are never safe.

How To Make Your Own ACV At Home: 7 Simple Steps

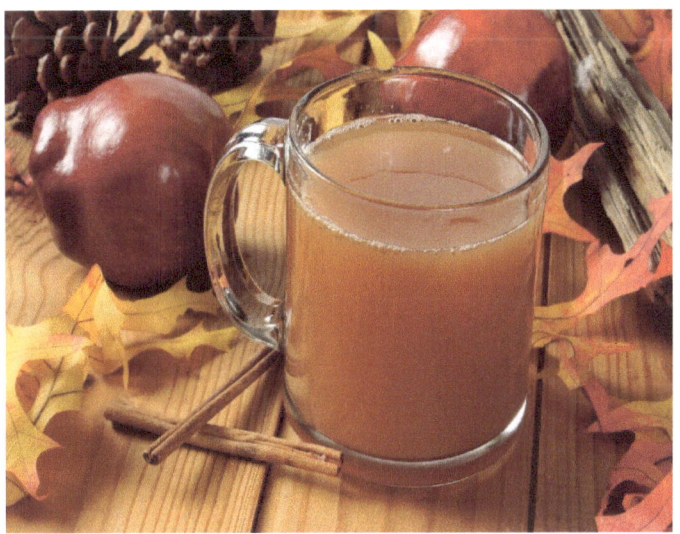

You can also make your own at home. Here are two simple ways you can use to make your own Apple Cider Vinegar at home. You will save yourself a trip to the store and quite some money.

Step 1: Wash and chop 10 apples into 1-inch cubes. Use only filtered water for the washing. If you are using scraps, it is okay, as well; you can keep the stems and seeds for this purpose.

Step 2: Take a one-gallon glass jar and fill it halfway with the cubed apples.

Step 3: Pour filtered water over the apples until the jar is at least 2/3rd full. The best ratio is – water, two parts and apples, one part.

Step 4: Add sugar to the mix; for every quart of water add 1/4th cup sugar. Use only organic honey or organic cane sugar. Mix thoroughly with a wooden spoon and continue mixing off and on for about an hour.

Keep the jar covered with cheesecloth. Do this every day for one week. Keep the jar in a warm and dark place.

Expect to see foaming and bubbling. This means that fermentation is taking place. You will also observe a strong, pungent smell. The apples, in due course, will settle at the bottom.

Step 5: Remove the apples after they have settled at the bottom. Strain them through the cheesecloth. Keep only the liquid. Close the mouth of the jar with cheesecloth.

Step 6: Place the glass jar and store again as previously. From now onwards, no stirring is required. You will need to keep the jar like this for about 4-6 weeks, in which time the mother will form and become visible on the surface of the liquid.

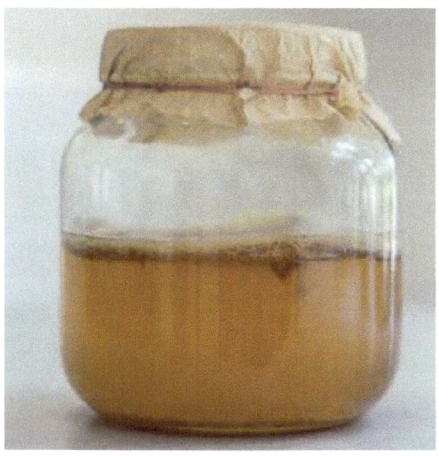

Step 7: Seal the jar with a lid and keep for another two weeks without disturbing it. During this period, the alcohol content of the liquid will be lost and will turn acidic. Your ACV is now ready for use.

How to Make ACV from Throwaway Ingredients?

You need not worry about money when you want an excellent quality apple cider vinegar. You can make it out of scraps, and this will cost you next to nothing while you will get an excellent quality ACV. Check out this process, which anyone can do, anywhere, anytime.

You will need the following **ingredients:**

- Cores and peels of 6-8 apples (The peels should be retained after they have been washed thoroughly. They should be collected from exclusively organic apples.)

- Large jar (one-quart size)

- One canning lid or rubber band

- Coffee filter

- Granulated sugar – 2½ tablespoons (You can substitute it with raw honey. You can also do without the sugar altogether. In that case the fermentation will be a little slower.)

- Boiled and cooled water – 2 ½ cups

It's okay if the peels are from bruised apples or have become brown. However, do not use peels from rotten apples or those which have developed mould.

In case you are using a glass jar of any other size, it's okay. Keep in mind the ratio of water to sugar – for every 1 cup of water you need to add 1 tablespoon of sugar.

Method:

- Place all the apple scraps into the glass jar, filling it up to three-quarters.

- Add 2 cups of water (the apples should be completely submerged) and 2 tablespoons of sugar. It is very important to ensure that the apple scraps are submerged because the exposed parts usually develop mould.

If required, use a wood stick or cap inside the jar to keep the apples submerged.

- Stir the mix well and cover with a coffee filter. Fix it with the help of a rubber band or a canning band.

- Place in dark and warm place for two weeks. [Don't forget about it.] After two weeks, you will observe that the liquid froths and has bubbles, which means that it has started the fermentation process.

- Strain the apple scraps out and retain the liquid. Cover with a coffee filter and store again. After one 1-2 weeks, the liquid will become cloudy and develop a spider-web on the surface. This is the mother, which will tell you that your ACV is ready.

- Keep tasting it every week until you find it suitable to your preference. At that time remove the coffee filter and close with a lid – which will stop the fermentation process.

- Place the ACV in the refrigerator and use as you require.

Properties of (Organic) Apple Cider Vinegar

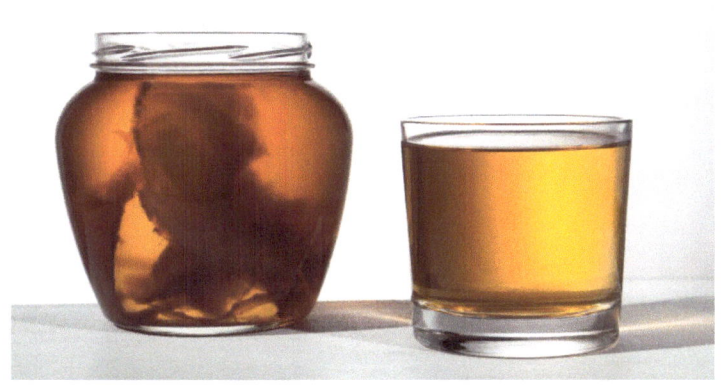

You wonder why there is so much talk about ACV? Check out a few of the top properties for which it is revered not only today but even some 5,000 years ago in the ancient civilizations of the world.

Anti-diabetic Properties

ACV through its compound – acetic acid – has an anti-glycemic effect. The effect is perhaps caused by the ability of acetic acid to inhibit the total digestion of carbohydrates. This in turn prevents blood sugar spiking.

Studies show that ACV can enhance insulin sensitivity by 19 per cent in Type-II diabetics and in pre-diabetics by 34 per cent.

Antimicrobial Properties

ACV is a powerful microbicide. Studies show that the organic acids it contains are potent enough to kill the dreaded E. coli bacteria as well as salmonella. Some of the organic acids that need mentioning here are tartaric acid, succinic acid, propionic acid, malic acid, citric acid, ascorbic acid, lactic acid and acetic acid.

Antioxidant Properties

Effective in neutralizing bad cholesterol levels	
Aids in restoring glow of skin	Helps to prevent cancer
Beneficial for maintaining proper blood glucose levels	
Speeds up the metabolism of body	Helps to cleanse entire digestive system
Useful in dandruff control and balancing pH level of scalp	
Relieves pain in joints and curbs progress of arthritis	Excellent therapy for losing excess weight
Helps to treat diarrhea symptoms by forming bulk fibrous matter	

Antioxidant agents such as chlorogenic acid, caffeic, gallic, epicatechin, and catechin are what give the ACV its antioxidant properties. It not only prevents rapid oxidisation that is normally caused by free-radicals in your body, but also reverses ageing symptoms to a large extent. You will find that ACV is often referred to as the "fountain of youth" in old and ancient records.

Brain Health Properties

Some studies have shown that ACV through sphingolipids (a precursor that helps repair and regenerate brain tissue) is able to enhance cognitive brain functions.

Digestive Properties

Reflux or heartburn is often the result of too little and NOT too much acid in your stomach; contrary to common beliefs. The ACV adds power to the acid in the stomach and almost instantly you lose that burning sensation.

Fighting Cancer

Owing to its high anti-oxidant content, organic vinegar is an excellent anti-cancer compound. It might not always reverse the disease, but it has the ability to slow it from advancing. It is also an excellent preventive for cancer and cancer-related ailments.

Heart Health Properties

The ACV components have the ability to lower and/ or eliminate almost all the factors that could affect the health of your heart. It lowers blood pressure, levels of cholesterol while at the same time keeping the arteries and other vital blood vessels clean and supple.

Increases Assimilation of Nutrients

The one ingredient that keeps popping up in all the benefits that ACV provides is the acetic acid. This component has the ability to improve assimilation of all the nutrients, especially minerals that are locked in the ingested foods.

Weight-Loss Aid

ACV has the ability of enhancing the satiation point; hence, helping reduce the quantity of food required per day. In other words, ACV helps reduce the amount of food you eat simply by making you feel full quicker and longer.

Warning: What You Need to Know When You Use ACV

This is an amazing food. However, there are a few "ifs" and "buts" that you need to consider when you decide to bring this amazing product into your daily life.

High Acid Content

Vinegar is highly acidic in nature. This means it has a horribly strong and pungent taste that very rarely can be consumed raw. It is a good idea to dilute it with a little water. It is NOT advisable to take ACV raw (undiluted) as it can damage your teeth enamel and even burn your throat.

Side Effects of Excessive Use

Excessive use of ACV may actually be harmful rather than helpful. Normally, ACV has the ability to increase the level of potassium in the body – a key mineral for many processes of the human body – which means it can improve, memory, heart health and bone density.

It is highly recommended that you ALWAYS consult a doctor before you make any drastic changes in your life; particularly, when it can impact your health in so many ways.

Interaction with Medicines

ACV may and could interact with medication for heart problems and diabetes. It could also interfere with laxatives and diuretics. If you are under any medication, inform your doctor before using ACV therapeutically.

Chapter 2: ACV As A Health Remedy

Apple Cider Vinegar is an elixir for good health. There are so many benefits that this modest liquid can bring to your life.

Potassium Deficiency

Some of the signs that you are suffering from potassium deficiency are:

- Lower back pain; joints, muscles and bone pain

- Fatigue; easily tired when faced with any type of mental or physical effort

- Headaches

- Lackluster hair; often looks like straw

- Dry scalp, dandruff, hair fall, balding

- Itchy eyes, look bloodshot

- Difficulty in focusing

- Low mental alertness

- Easily irritable and depressed

- Cold hands and feet – even in warm weather – could be a sign of potassium deficiency as well

- Diseases such as atherosclerosis, lupus, Crohn's disease, multiple sclerosis, Alzheimer's disease, IBS (irritable bowel syndrome), hypothyroidism, ulcerative colitis, coronary artery disease, high blood pressure, celiac disease, adrenal insufficiency, atrial fibrillation, kidney stones and arthritis are caused by lack of potassium.

A very rich source of potassium, ACV helps where potassium does not easily come from daily diet. Potassium is one of the essential nutrients that are required to maintain the health of tissues (repair and regeneration) including teeth, nails and bones.

Growth And Development

Potassium is also one of the key ingredients for growth. Children who are potassium deficient are slow developers and do not grow as they should according to their age. Just a few teaspoons of ACV every day can work miracles. Potassium also calms people who are prone to anxiety attacks.

Anti-Ageing For Both Mind And Body

To regain a youthful appearance, to grow well, to maintain the health of your hair, nails, teeth and bones – you need potassium. You can have this amazing mineral from ACV, for which reason this vinegar is also known as the elixir of youth or the "fountain of youth".

Experimental studies that involved introducing ACV in the diet of senile senior persons brought about amazing results. The senile senior persons not only regained their energy and younger looking skin, but also their mental abilities.

Heart Health

Potassium is also a most powerful cleaner of the arteries. It removes all the residue build-up from unhealthy eating habits and lifestyle. Owing to this property, potassium is nicknamed as the "detergent of the arteries".

Energy Tonic

Mix into a regular glass of water 2 teaspoons of ACV and 2 spoons of raw honey. Drink it at once or sip it like tea. This will relieve chronic physical fatigue, body ache and muscle stiffness.

Weight-Loss Aid

Use ACV to lose weight. Use the ACV mix – 1 teaspoon raw honey, 1 teaspoon ACV (honey and ACV should always be in 1:1 ratio) in a glass of water. Take this mix 3 times a day and ensure that your daily calorie intake is 1,200.

Another potent mix against body fat is 3 parts ACV and 1-part virgin olive oil. Use this as a daily massage solution for elimination of fat under the skin and skin toning.

Detoxification

ACV is an excellent detoxification agent. The mother enzyme found in ACV is a powerful detox agent that can neutralize and eliminate most toxins from the body through a process that scientists call *"acetolysis"*.

Use the ACV mix described earlier (1 teaspoon each raw honey and ACV in a glass of water). In addition to that, you could try juice made of 1 teaspoon of ACV and 6 oz of fresh vegetables (tomatoes/carrots and greens) in between your meals.

Cures Headaches and Migraines

There are two major types or categories of headaches, i.e. the emotional type and those triggered by physical illness. The physical types are the result of some or other imbalance caused by a toxic build-up in the body. The emotional headaches are the result of emotional problems – fear, stress, irritation, etc.

You can get rid of commercial and OTC painkillers used for this purpose. ACV balances the pH of the body and helps by alkalizing it. Diseases cannot exist in an alkaline environment. ACV also has the ability to calm anxiety and nervousness and restore mental alertness. Daily use of ACV will ensure that the headaches will reduce and ultimately disappear.

You can use ACV for inhalation, as well – this will clear the sinuses quicker and relieve the pain. Place 2 tablespoons of ACV and 2 cups of water in a vaporizer or saucepan. Inhale the vapors 5-10 times taking in deep breaths.

Combine this with ACV compress to the head and shoulders where muscles tend to get tense owing to stress and anxiety.

Mouth and Throat Care

Sore Throat

Have a bad sore throat and need quick relief and no medication healing? Take half-a-glass of water and add to it 1 teaspoon of ACV. Gargle with this mix three times consecutively every alternate hour. This will kill the harmful germs and relieve the pain.

Mouth Freshener & Hygiene

Used as mouthwash, ACV mix fights plaque, removes tartar and kills harmful bacteria in the mouth. It also promotes healing of gum diseases and fights bad breath.

Whitening of Teeth

You can keep your pearly whites sparkling and stain free with ACV. Make a solution of ACV and water in 1:2 ratio. Swish this solution around your teeth for about 1 minute, then brush as usual.

You can also clean your dentures with ACV. Soak the dentures in 1:1 ACV and water solution; brush well in the morning.

Healthy Skin

Skin Infections

- **Herpes (Cold Sores and Genital Sores)** – Apply ACV directly to the affected area to have it heal quickly. It immediately relieves the pain, discomfort and itchiness.

- **Poison Ivy and Insect Bites** – ACV instantly reduces inflammation, disinfects and reduces itchiness. Keep the ACV mix refrigerated for best results.

- **Bruises and Wounds** – excellent disinfectant, ACV can be used for minor bruises, cuts and burns. It helps blood clot on open wounds as well as fights infection. For quick relief, soak a cotton ball in ACV and apply to the spot directly.

- **Varicose veins** – use undiluted ACV and have a towel soaked in it. Wrap towel on the affected parts every night. Gently massage ACV in the affected areas as well. In the meantime, you should consume the ACV mix every day.

- **Fungal Infection** – one of the most stubborn infections, fungal infections have a knack of recurring again and again, ACV is excellent for this.

- Use 1:1 mix of ACV and distilled water for athlete's foot, jock itch, eczema. Soak the part with the lukewarm mix

- For thrush and sore throat, gargle every 2-3 hours, three times consecutively with a mix of 1 teaspoon ACV and 1 cup warm water.

- For diaper rash, genital area yeast infections, apply cotton ball soaked in a mix of 1 tablespoon ACV and 1-quart water to the area for at least 10 days consecutively.

Digestive System

Digestion problems can be eliminated with the help of ACV. Just before your meals, take ½ teaspoon of ACV and swirl in the mouth for approximately 30 secs to 1 minute; then swallow. This will promote the production of saliva and stimulate digestive juices in the stomach.

Kidney and Urinary Bladder

If you are prone to kidney and/ or urinary bladder problems, use ACV in your daily diet regularly, three times a day. Also, ensure that you drink enough water – at least 8 glasses per day, every day. In addition to the ACV drink, you could try adopting a watermelon only diet for 3 days once in every 6 months. During these days, you should eat nothing but watermelon – including the seeds. This not only cleanses but also heals kidneys and bladder.

Kidney/ Gall Bladder Cleansing

Make this mix to cleanse the kidneys and gall bladder; you need to do this twice a year or once a year. Take the following ingredients to make a mix:

- ½ teaspoon of ACV

- 1 teaspoon of buckwheat honey

- 2 tablespoons dried/ fresh corn silk

- 1 quart distilled water (you can also use herbal tea)

Drink 1 cup of this mix three times a day for 1 month.

Bedwetting

This is excellent for children who cannot stop bedwetting. Mix 1 teaspoon of buckwheat honey with ½ teaspoon ACV and administer at night before bed. The child should not have any water for at least 3 hours before bedtime.

Kidney/ Gall Bladder Stones Two-Day Flush

Before starting this process, you need to prepare your body about one week in advance. Start by drinking a mix of ½ teaspoon ACV in a glass of apple juice (6 oz). This is not advisable for diabetics.

The apple juice is a rich source of enzymes, pectin, potassium and malic acid, which cleanse the body and soften the stones, making it easy to dissolve and remove from the body. You need to do this twice a year to ensure that you flush out all the stones and prevent this from becoming a painful problem.

The two-day flush process needs to follow the steps described below:

Day No 1: Take a large glass that can contain 8 oz. Mix 1/3 Extra Virgin Olive Oil and 2/3 Organic Apple Juice. To this mix add 1 teaspoon Organic Apple Cider Vinegar.

Drink this mix in an 8 oz glass three times on the first day. If you are hungry, you can have as much apple juice as you want, but no water, other liquid or food; nothing else. At night, make it a point to sleep on the right side with your knee pulled up towards your chest. This helps the flushing process.

Day No 2: On the second day, drink the ACV mix only twice; once morning and once at night. Have as much apple juice as you want, but no water, other liquid or food; nothing else. Sleep the same way as the first night.

Day No 3: On the third day, start eating midday (11 a.m. onwards). Start with a raw salad made with lettuce, sprouts, tomatoes, celery, carrots, and cabbage seasoned with extra virgin olive oil and ACV; you may also season with brewer's yeast and coriander.

Continue eating this the whole day. You may also have (lightly) steamed vegetables such as leafy greens, chard, collards, and kale.

The stones will be expelled through the stool. If you check, you will see a number of greenish or brown pellets of various sizes in your stool.

You need to do this twice a year to ensure that your body is detoxified and stays free of stones and toxins.

IMPORTANT: *Since this is a detoxification process, you might feel nauseous and sick. Do not worry; this means that the detox is working just fine. When you feel sick, drink 2-3 glasses of water and throw up. You will feel okay instantly.*

Enlarged Prostate

Make a salad dressing mix out of the 2 tablespoons of ACV, 2 tablespoons of olive oil, a dash of cinnamon and a little Braggs Liquid Aminos. Use this salad dressing on raw and steamed vegetables. You will also need zinc, which you can get from raw pumpkin seeds. Be liberal with the seeds; they taste good and are good for you as well.

You will also benefit from adding Saw Palmetto, Prostex and Zinc health supplements.

Health Benefits for Women

The ACV is an excellent tonic for the vagina, as well. It helps keep infection away by balancing the pH. The ACV and the vagina's optimal pH is the same.

Douche Mix with ACV

Take 2 quarts of distilled water and add to it 2 tablespoons of ACV. Use this once a week or twice a month to ensure that no infection affects you. If you suffer from a yeast infection or have any type of discharge, apply 1-2 times a day until the infection is gone and the discharge lessens.

ACV for Menopausal Hot Flushes

Hot flushes are among the most annoying symptoms of menopausal women. You can get rid of them by drinking the ACV solution 3-5 times a day over 6 months to one year. Besides eliminating hot flushes, you will enjoy all the other benefits that regular intake of ACV offers.

Diagnosing Cervical Cancer with ACV

Research carried out by the John Hopkins University has shown that cervical cancer can be diagnosed very easily – and what is important, very accurately – with the help of ACV. All you need to do is swab the cervix with ACV. If it is cancerous, the area will turn completely white. This test is much quicker, much cheaper than the PAP smear. Being affordable, it is a great thing for developing countries and people who have problems with funds.

Arthritis Treatment

Arthritis can be prevented and reversed with the help of ACV. Make an ACV drink with 2 teaspoons of ACV and 2 teaspoons of raw organic honey in 8 oz of water. Drink this one hour before your meals (lunch/ dinner) every day. The hard deposits that cause pain and inflammation in the joints will be flushed out. You will regain the flexibility of the joints; inflammation and pain will also go.

In addition to the ACV mix, you will do well to ensure the following:

- Drink at least 8 glasses of distilled water.

- Try to ensure that 60-70 per cent of the food on your plate is raw and organic.

- Take health supplements such as cod liver oil (2 teaspoons), alfalfa tablets, MSM combo, chondroitin sulfates, glucosamine, multi-vitamin and minerals.

Cold Cure

Mix in a cup ¼ cup of honey with a ¼ cup of Apple Cider Vinegar. Administer 2 teaspoons 4-8 times daily for 3-5 days. All the symptoms of the cold will disappear.

ACV Is Great for Animals

Clean Great Fur

Mix 1 cup ACV with 3 cups of filtered water and store in a jar. Give 1 teaspoon of this mix to small animals and 2-3 teaspoons to large animals. The animals will grow beautiful fur, stay healthy and energetic.

Skin Infections

- Apply the diluted ACV to the skin to treat itching (from

infections) and rashes. If the animal has lice and/ or fleas, rinse with ACV.

- Add a little (1 teaspoon to 1-quart water) ACV to your pet's drinking water to keep away mange.

Calms Down Chicken

If you are growing chicken, you know how difficult it is to control chickens fighting and how infectious it is. Once they start pecking one another, it becomes a total mayhem. Just add a little ACV (1 teaspoon to 1-quart water) to their drinking water, and they will be calm and happy.

Chapter 3: ACV as A Beauty Aid

Apple Cider Vinegar can be used as a beauty aid remedy for a number of conditions. It is affordable, it is extremely effective, and you can even make it at home – so it is available anytime you want it.

Youthful Skin

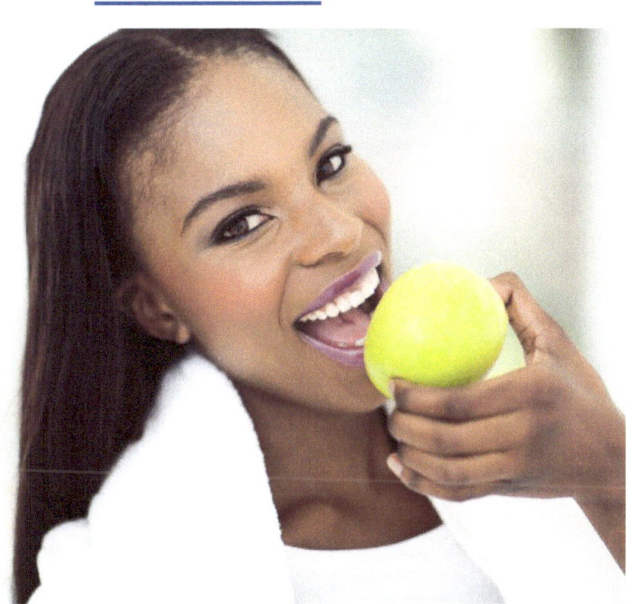

Cleaning And Detoxifying Skin

Use the ACV skin massage to enjoy a most vibrant healthy and youthful look. Mix ½ cup of ACV with 4 cups of warm distilled water. Rub this water all over your skin and massage gently until your body dries off completely. This balances the pH of the skin and also draws out (detoxifies) toxins through the skin – one of the most powerful and quickest ways to detoxify and feel great.

Use ACV in place of soap; use a loofah to remove dead skin cells. Within no time, you will feel the skin healthier, and others will see it. Your skin will feel soft, fresh and toned.

Toning Skin

For further toning of the skin, steam your face with an ACV mix of 1 quart of distilled water to which 3 tablespoons of ACV have been added. Further, rub a cotton ball dipped in the ACV solution to clean the surface of the skin. Repeat steaming; then remove blackheads. To close skin pores, refrigerate a mix of 1:1 ACV and distilled water. Spray this mix all over the face for instant skin tightening.

Repeat this process twice a week to enjoy a flawless, smooth and youthful looking skin.

Natural Face Lift

Wash your face with cold water – no soap. Mix ACV and distilled water in 1:1 proportion in a small basin. Apply a hot towel to the face for about 3 minutes and remove. Soak a towel in the ACV mix, wring loosely and then apply to the face. Place the hot towel over the ACV soaked towel and keep it on the face for 3-5 minutes and remove.

Once again, apply the ACV soaked towel on the face and lie down with feet elevated for about 10 minutes. Gently scrub the face with the towel. Rinse with cold water. Repeat this twice a week; it will take 10 years off your face.

Sunburn Remedy

Dip cotton in undiluted ACV and pat on the affected skin. Do not wash away. This prevents blistering and reduces pain. You can also soak in a tub of room-temperature water to which 1-2 cups of ACV have been added. Soak for 15-20 minutes, come out of the water and pat dry. Apply aloe-vera gel to the affected areas.

Remove Warts from Skin

Make a mix of ACV and glycerin in equal measures. Apply to the warts by dabbing lightly. Do it 4-5 times a day until it dissolves completely.

Hair Care

ACV can be immensely helpful for hair problems.

Dandruff Cure

Dip cotton in undiluted ACV and tap it gently on the scalp, parting the hair while doing so to ensure that it reaches the scalp. After you have applied to the whole scalp, wrap hair with a hot towel and leave on until the towel is cold. Wash as you would normally with shampoo. The ACV restores the pH of the skin, removes dryness and infections. The result is sparkling clean scalp with no dandruff.

Dry Hair

- Apply ACV to the scalp and castor oil to the hair and wrap with a hot towel. Leave it on for at least 30 minutes. Wash with shampoo. Repeat every week.

- Use a mix of 1/3 cup of ACV and 1 quart of water as the last rinse for your hair. This will ensure that dandruff stays away and also gives your hair a stunning shine.

Hair Fall/ Balding Problem

- Mix 2 tablespoons of ACV in a cup of water and add to it one pinch of cayenne powder. Apply this mix to the scalp about half-an-hour before you shampoo.

- Make a mix of Acv and royal jelly in 1:1 proportion. Apply on the spot to the balding areas. Leave it to dry overnight. Wash off the next day as you would normally do with shampoo.

Deodorant

Underarms

ACV kills bacteria and it is bacteria that causes body odor. To enjoy a low-cost, highly-effective deodorant, dab a little ACV under your arm and let it dry before you wear your clothes. The smell will go as it mixes with that of your body; at the same time, it will prevent the formation of body odor.

Crotch Area

You can also dab ACV on the crotch for the same reason. It prevents bacteria from forming in this region and creating rashes and bad odor. ACV takes care of body hygiene and body odor.

Feet Odor

Soak your feet in a solution of ACV and water (ration 1:3). Alternatively, you can dab your feet with undiluted ACV. Let it dry. Wear socks and shoes as usual. This not only prevents feet odor, but it also prevents fungal infection, Athlete's foot, and nail fungus.

Chapter 4: ACV Uses As A Natural Cleaner

ACV is indeed primarily known as a health boon for humanity. However, it is also an excellent organic cleaner. It has an amazing range of uses outside the therapeutic use. One among these uses is as a cleaning agent, which is also affordable, available and extremely effective.

Prevents and Absorbs Bad Odor

- You can place ACV in a bowl in the corner of each room to ensure that it does not develop bad odor – especially in rooms that stay closed for a long time.

- You can also put a bowl in your refrigerator to ensure that no odor will spread in the refrigerator.

- Remove odor (and grease) from dishes by adding 2 teaspoons of ACV to the hot detergent water. You can achieve the same goal by wiping the fridge with a solution of 1:1 vinegar and water.

- Remove the odor from the wooden cutting board by wiping it with undiluted ACV. This will also kill all the bacteria and harmful organisms, making it safe to use.

- Deodorize jars for instant use, using a rinse of vinegar. You can reuse mayonnaise, mustard and what-not jars immediately.

- Lunch box smelling of yesterday's food? Soak a slice of bread in ACV and close it in the lunch box. Leave closed for

15-30 minutes; open, and the smell will be gone.

- Make your own air freshener/ air purifier by spraying the room/ area with undiluted vinegar. The vinegar will absorb all the smells and leave behind an amazingly fresh smell and feel.

- Deodorize your shoes by spraying the inside with vinegar and then refrigerating it overnight in a paper bag.

Removes Fruit Stains From Skin

Rub hand with undiluted ACV. Leave on until it dries. Rub again and then rinse with water.

Aquarium Glass Cleaner

You can eliminate the water stains left on the glass in your aquarium. Dip a small piece of cotton in undiluted vinegar and rub the glass with it. Leave for a few hours. Rinse with water.

Milking Equipment Cleaner

Milk spoils easily if it comes into contact with any bacteria or chemicals. Hence, it is important that the milk equipment is kept clean. Use undiluted ACV for cleaning the equipment. You will have clean, bacteria free and odorless apparatus.

Digital Equipment

Wipe the surface of your digital equipment – computer, mobile phone, tablet – with a solution of 1:1 ACV and water. They'll be shiny again in no time.

Cleans Rust

- Take your rusty implement or tool and soak it in undiluted

ACV overnight. Wipe clean.

- This formula also works with the car chrome parts. Use undiluted vinegar.

- You can use a cloth soaked in vinegar to wipe stainless steel to get an amazing good as new glaze.

Clean Washing Machine

Add 1 cup of vinegar to the water load in the machine and run the machine through a normal cycle (without any clothes). This will get rid of the soap scum from the hoses and freshen the machine up for you.

Unclog Items

- **Steam Iron** – Make a mix of an equal quantity of ACV and water and pour into the steam chamber of the iron. Plug in to iron, fix it to the steam setting and leave it on for 5-10 minutes. Unplug and let it cool. When it cools down, remove the water from the chamber. All the impurities will come away with the water.

- **Kitchen Drain** – pour ½ cup of baking soda down the drain. Follow it with ½ cup of ACV. Pour 5-6 cups of boiling water.

Remove Stains

- If you are cooking on a plate, you know how unsightly it will look when it is burnt. You can get rid of the burn marks by heating a mix of equal parts of vinegar and salt. Allow to cool and wipe; stains will be gone.

- If your China is stained, the same mix will clear the tea and coffee stains.

- Removes hard water stains. Soak a cloth in undiluted ACV and wipe the hard water lines. Leave overnight. Clean the next morning.

- ACV shines pewter, copper and brass when polished with a mix of 1 cup ACV and 1 teaspoon of salt.

- Use full-strength ACV to remove ink stains from the walls and floors. If you have young children, you will appreciate this tip very much.

- Remove mildew stains from your shower curtain by washing it in the washing machine along with 2 cups of vinegar. Wash only the shower curtain; don't add any clothes.

- Remove stains from wood by rubbing undiluted vinegar over it. For a super polish finish, take 2 cups of water and mix with ¼ vinegar and 2 tablespoons olive oil. Polish the wood until it shines.

Silver Polish

Add 2 tablespoons baking soda to ½ cup vinegar and mix well. Place all your silverware in the mix and set aside for about 2 hours. Remove from the mix and place in cold water; wipe dry immediately and store in a dry place.

Chapter 5: Other Uses Of Apple Cider Vinegar

Frost-Free Car Windshield

Wipe the glass inside and out with a solution of vinegar (3 parts) and water (1 part). Leave overnight. The next day, the glass will not be affected by frost.

Gardener's Friend

Killer of Weeds

Mix 1-part vinegar and 3 parts water and spray over weeds; this is a natural weed killer – totally natural and non-toxic.

Killer of Mold

You can ensure that your pumpkins and melons stay free of mold – that tend to develop on their skin owing to the humidity and proximity to the earth – by spraying undiluted ACV on the vegetables every alternate day.

Bathroom Cleaner

All Surfaces

You can have a sparkling and bacteria free bathroom by using ACV as a cleaner. Use vinegar to wipe all surfaces to prevent and remove mildew marks. This will deodorize the bathroom and clean all stains.

Showerheads

Soak the showerhead in diluted vinegar solution overnight. Unscrew it if possible; if not, wrap a soaked-in-vinegar cloth around it overnight.

Great Trick For Painters

Before starting to paint on canvas, wipe the whole canvas with a cotton ball soaked in vinegar. This will not only wipe all the dirt, grime and micro-debris from the canvas, but also disinfect it. In this way, the paint will adhere better and look brighter.

Cooking Tricks Using ACV

Freshen Up Vegetables

Are your vegetables a little wilted? Make a mix of 2 cups of (room temperature) water with 2 teaspoons of salt. Soak the vegetables for 30 minutes in it. They will suddenly look bright and fresh – and as appetizing as ever.

Tenderize Meat

Add ACV to the meat – ¼ cup per 3 lb. meat – and leave overnight. Remember to add your favorite herbs to the marinade so it permeates the meat. Cook without rinsing or draining the vinegar.

Gelatin Trick

Add 1 teaspoon of ACV per box of gelatin to firm the dessert up, even when it is hot. It will resist sagging and look superb.

Lemon Substitute

Forgot to buy a lemon and you need it for the dish you are preparing? Don't panic; use ¼ teaspoon of ACV for every lemon you would have used.

Instant Buttermilk

Need buttermilk instant? You can make it using 1 cup of milk and 2 teaspoons of ACV. Let it set for 5-10 minutes then enjoy

.

Worms And Bugs?

Are the vegetables you got worrying you? Dip the vegetables in a quick solution of vinegar and salt. No sooner you do that the bugs will fall out in the solution.

Fish Scaling

Rub undiluted ACV on the fish to get the scales off almost with no effort.

Melts Chicken Bones

Soak a chicken bone in undiluted vinegar for 3-4 days. The chicken bone will become as flexible as rubber. This is a great trick to know in time of need.

Fix Egg White In Water Poach

If you want perfect water-poach egg, add 2 tablespoons ACV to 1 cup of water when you are poaching the egg. The egg white will not bleed or spread.

Vegan Cake Trick

Mix baking soda with ACV as a rising agent for a vegan cake. It rises like magic.

Remove Glue

- Need to loosen glued joints of furniture around the house or tools? Spray undiluted vinegar to the joints and leave overnight.

- So many times you want to get rid of the label on the glass, shoes, phone cover, etc. and then realize that you are stuck with the glue, which is even more troublesome. Wipe it with cotton dipped in undiluted vinegar to get the glue to disappear.

ACV As Pest Control

Cat Repellant

Spray a little of diluted ACV (1 teaspoon in 1 cup) on the area where you do not want your cat to walk, climb or scratch. The smell will go away pretty soon for you but will stay on for the cat for a long time.

This is a great trick if you have both young children (who love to play in sand) and cats as pets who want to poop in the sand. Just spray vinegar all around the sand and the cat will stay away.

Ant Repellant

Spray diluted ACV (1 teaspoon in 1 cup) on the window sills and ant trails to prevent an ant attack.

Fly Trap

Fill a large jar halfway with Apple Cider Vinegar. Close the lid on it after you punch holes through it. The holes will be big enough to allow insects to go inside. The flies, attracted by the vinegar, will go through the holes, but will be unable to crawl back.

No More Urine Stains

Add ¼ teaspoon of ACV to the water bowl of your pet dog. The urine will no longer stain your lawn when he relieves himself.

Mosquito Repellant

Use undiluted vinegar to spray all the exposed parts of your skin. Allow it to dry; DO NOT wipe off. The smell will go away in about 30 minutes, but no mosquito will touch you through the night.

Chapter 6: Quick And Delicious Apple Recipes To Help You Make Your ACV

Sometimes, you wish you had some quick and tasty recipes using apples just so you could have enough raw material to make apple cider vinegar with the lowest possible cost. Here are some amazing recipes that are as easy as ABC to make and will give you enough raw material for your ACV.

Apples and Berry Sauce

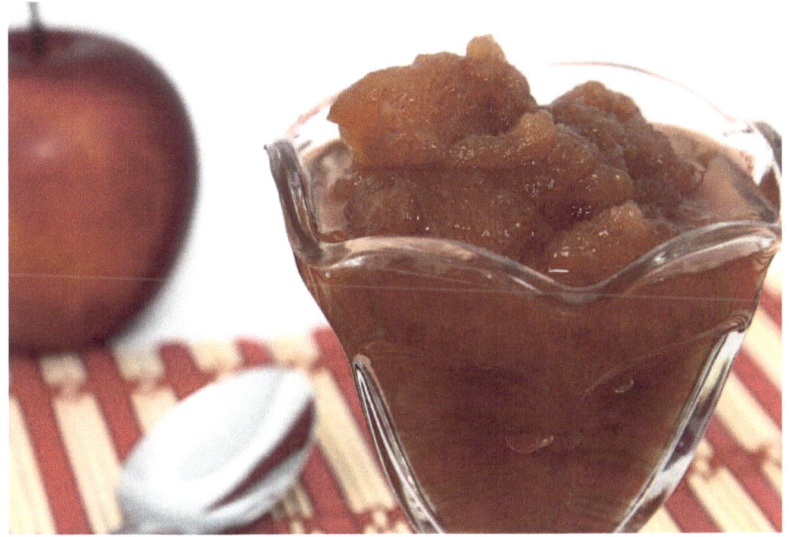

Ingredients:
- Apples – 1 lbs., deseeded, cored and chopped into 1-inch cubes
- Berries – ½ cup, frozen (anything you like or mixed)

- Orange juice – 1 tablespoon

- Raw honey – 1 tablespoon

Method:

- Place saucepan over medium heat and add all ingredients together. Stir often to mix and continue to heat until it bubbles.

- Reduce heat to a low simmer, cover partially and cook for 15 minutes. The apples should become soft – but not mushy.

- Remove from heat and place in a blender.

- Blend on low speed for about 20 seconds, for 2-3 minutes until totally smooth.

Homemade Fruit Butter Apple Vanilla

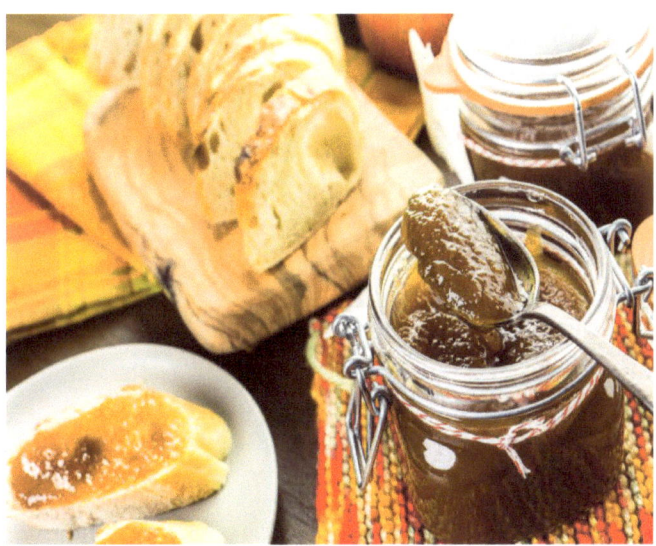

Ingredients:

- Apples – 3 lbs. chopped in 1-inch cubes

- Pears – 3 lbs. chopped in 1-inch cubes

- Maple syrup – 2 tablespoons

- Vanilla extract – 2 tablespoons

Method:

- Wash the fruits thoroughly

- Deseed, core and remove stems wherever necessary

- Place all the fruits in and cover.

- Cook on high heat for about 4-6 minutes. Reduce to low.

- Continue on low heat for a further 8 minutes.

- Transfer to a blender and blend until smooth. You can also use a hand blender.

- Return to cooking pot, with lid slightly open to allow the water to evaporate so the fruit butter thickens.

- Continue to cook for 2-6 hours until you get the consistency you desire.

- Allow to cool and place in glass jars. Refrigerate and use as you like.

Homemade Fruit Butter Apple Strawberry

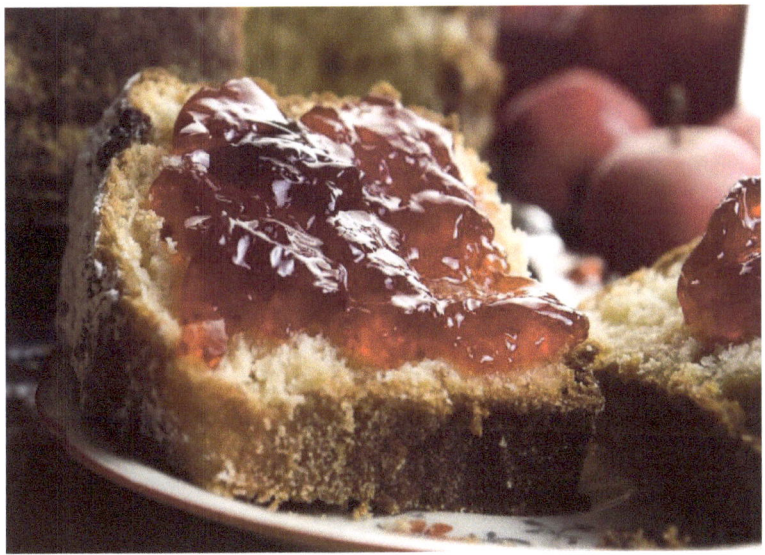

Ingredients:

- Apples – 3 lbs., cored, washed and chopped into 1-inch cubes

- Strawberry – 3 cups, washed

- Raw honey – ¼ cup (optional)

Method:

- Wash the fruits thoroughly

- Deseed remove stems wherever necessary

- Place all the fruits in a cooking pot and cover.

- Cook on low heat for about 12-16 minutes.

- Transfer to a blender and blend until smooth. You can also use a hand blender.

- Return to cooking pot, but this time let the lid slightly open to allow the water evaporate so the fruit butter thickens.

- Continue to cook on low heat for 2-6 hours until you get the consistency you desire.

- Allow to cool and place in glass jars. Refrigerate and use as you like.

Apple Oatmeal Breakfast Bar

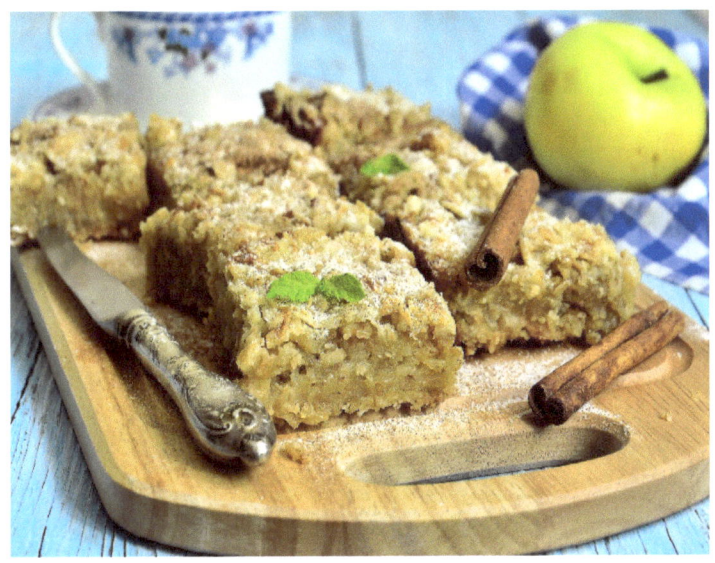

Ingredients:

- Apples – 2-3, washed, cored, peeled, diced into ¼ inch cubes

- Oat flour – ½ cup

- Whole wheat flour – 1 cup (or spelt flour)

- Raw honey – 3 tablespoons

- Salt – ½ teaspoon

- Baking soda – 1 teaspoon

- Baking powder – 1 teaspoon

- Cinnamon – 1½ teaspoon (or apple pie spice)

- Unsalted butter – 8 tablespoons (cold, cubed)

- Rolled oats – 1 cup

- Vanilla – 1 teaspoon

- Lemon juice – 1 teaspoon

Method:

- Butter 9"x9" baking dish

- Heat oven to 350 degrees

- Take a large bowl and mix in it the cinnamon, baking soda, baking powder, salt and flour.

- Add butter and honey and knead well until the whole mix is crumbly, moist and gathered in small pea-sized balls.

- Add oats and mix quickly. It is important that the butter does not melt in this process.

- Take 2 cup of this mix and place in the baking dish, spreading it on the bottom.

- Take 2 cups diced apples and place in a large (separate) bowl.

- Take the peels and the rest of what remained of the apples, add the lemon juice and vanilla and run through the blender until pureed to a smooth paste.

- Pour the puree over the diced apple in the large bowl and mix thoroughly.

- Pour this mix over the dry mix in the baking dish. Distribute the apple mix evenly and then pour the remaining flour mix over this. Press on it to make it a little tight.

- Bake it for about 30 minutes; the top will become golden brown.

- Allow to cool totally or it will crumble when cut.

- When cold, cut in the desired shape.

Apple cider vinegar salad dressing

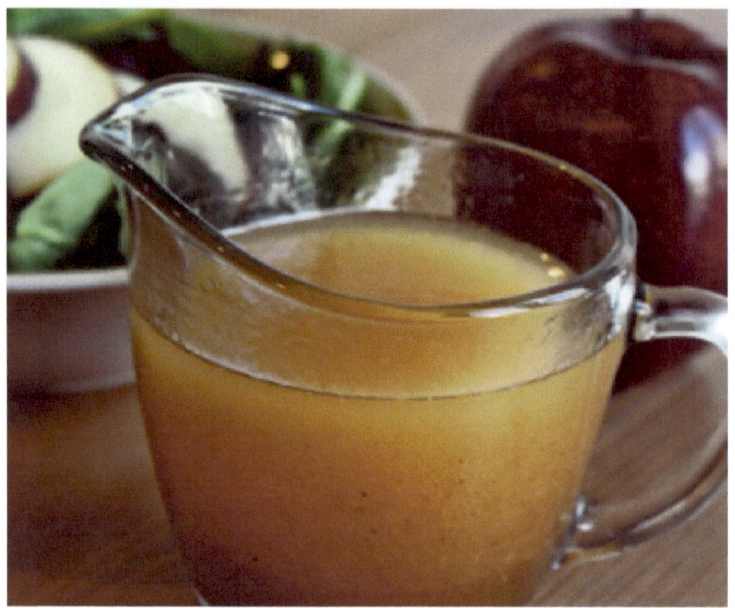

Preparation Time: 5 Min

Total Time: 5 Min

Ingredients:

- Shallot peeled, and cut, 1
- Olive oil: 1/3 cup
- Cider vinegar: ¼ cup
- Dijon mustard: 2 teaspoons
- Honey: 2 teaspoons
- Salt: ½ teaspoon
- Ground pepper: ¼ teaspoon

Method:

1. Blend all ingredients in a blender.

2. Pour the batter in an air tight jar then refrigerate for a week.

Nutritional Information:

- Calories: 13
- Fat: 0.5 g
- Carbs: 3 g
- Sugar: 2 g
- Sodium: 214 mg

Cider Vinegar Chicken

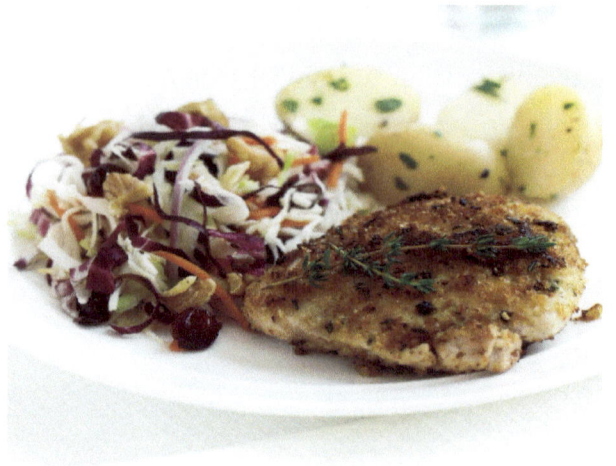

Serves: 6

Ingredients:

- Boneless chicken breasts: 6

- Garlic salt: 5 teaspoons

- Cider vinegar: 1 cup

- Breadcrumbs ½ cup

Method:

1. Preheat oven at 350 F.

2. Place chicken breasts onto a baking dish and pour over vinegar, sprinkle with salt, garlic and breadcrumbs.

3. Bake for 35 minutes.

Nutritional Information:

- Calories: 141 kcal

- Fat: 2.8 g

- Carbs: 0.9g

- Protein: 24.6 g

- Cholesterol: 67 mg

- Sodium: 1571 mg

Apple Cider Vinegar Braised Chicken Thighs

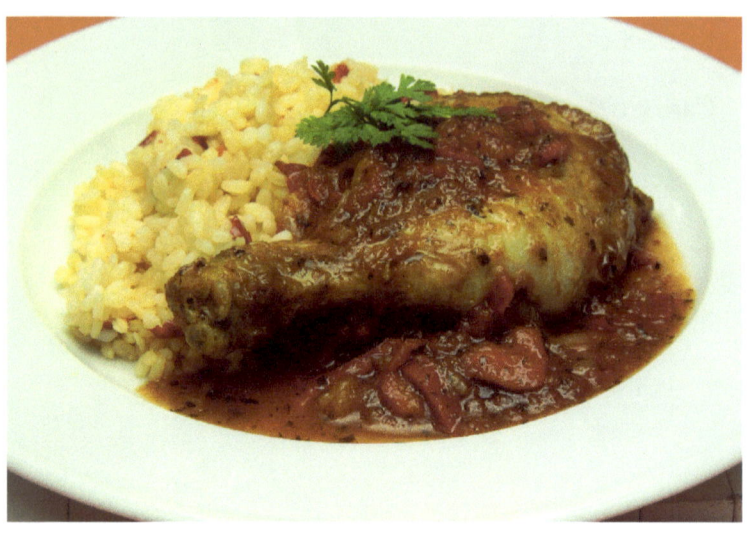

Preparation Time: 10 Min

Total Time: 1 Hr. 15 Min

Serves: 2

Ingredients:

- Olive Oil: 1 tablespoon.

- Chicken thighs: 4

- Salt and Pepper

- Carrots, sliced: 2

- Tomatoes, chopped 2

- Garlic, minced: 3 cloves

- Leek, sliced: 1

- Flour: 1 tablespoon.

- Apple Cider Vinegar: 1/2 cup

- Chicken Stock: 1-1/2 cups

- Butter: 1 tablespoon.

Method:

1. Preheat oven at 350 F.

2. Take a pot and heat olive oil.

3. Season thighs with salt and pepper then cook for 8-10 minutes. Set aside.

4. Now add garlic, leek, tomatoes and carrots, cook for 5 minutes.

5. Stir in flour, vinegar and chicken stock. Boil. and add chicken.

6. Cover pot and place in oven. Cook for 40 minutes.

7. Heat your broiler, remove chicken from pot to broiler pan. Broil for 6 minutes.

8. Return to stove on a low heat and add butter. Then serve.

Nutritional Information:

- 159 calories

- Fat 1 g

- Sodium 25 mg

- Protein 2 g

- Carbohydrate 40 g

- Sugar 26 g

- Fiber 4 g

- Iron 1 mg

- Calcium 38 mg

Zingy Cranberry Cocktail

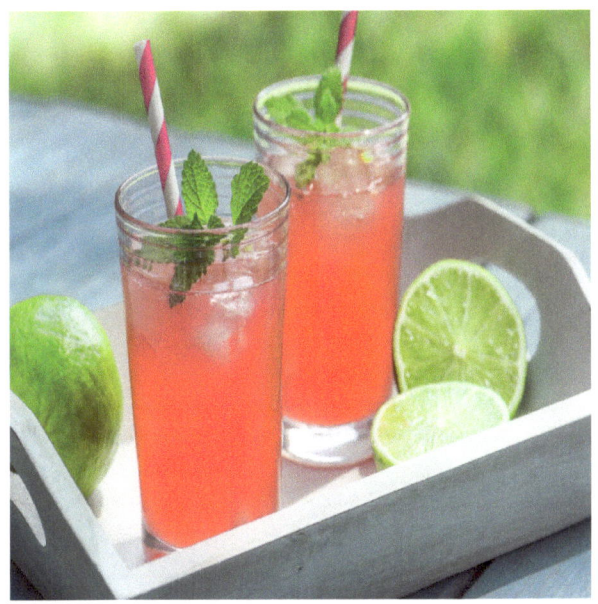

Preparation Time: 5 Min

Serves: 2

Ingredients:

- Apple cider vinegar: 1-2 tablespoons.

- Cranberry Juice: 2 tablespoons.

- Water: 2 ½ cups.

- Maple syrup: 2 teaspoons.

Method:

Mix all ingredients together and serve.

Nutritional Information:

Contains antioxidants.

Sweet Blaster

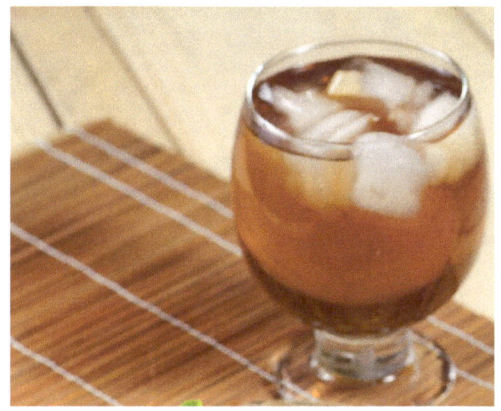

Preparation Time: 5 Min

Serves: 1

Ingredients:

- Water: 1 1/2 cups.

- Apple cider vinegar: 1-2 tablespoons.

- Black strap molasses: 2 teaspoons.

Method:

1. Mix all ingredients together and serve.

Nutritional Information:

Contains iron, calcium, magnesium and manganese.

Tomato Cider Slinger

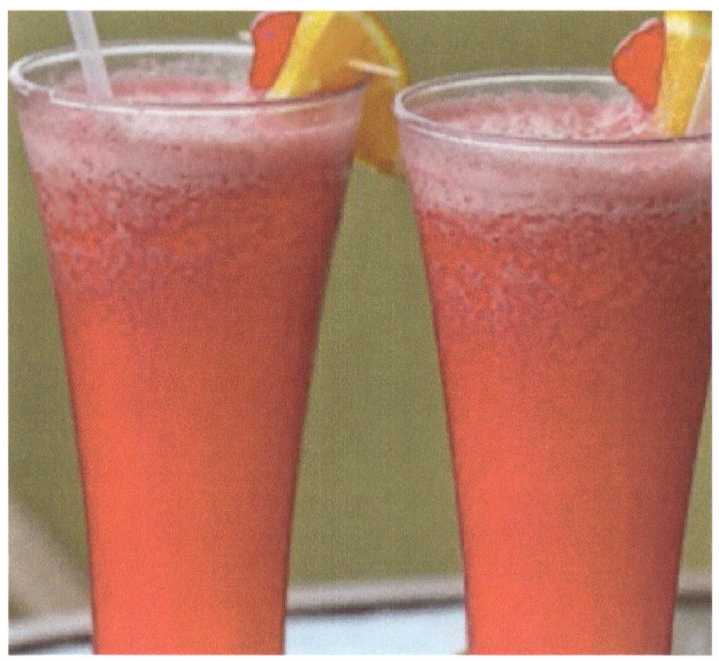

Preparation Time: 5 Min

Serves: 2

Ingredients:

- Tomato juice: 2 ½ cups.

- Apple cider vinegar: 2-3 tablespoons

- Sea salt: ½ teaspoon

Method:

1. Blend together all ingredients in a blender and serve.

Nutritional Information:

Contains antioxidants.

Super Juice

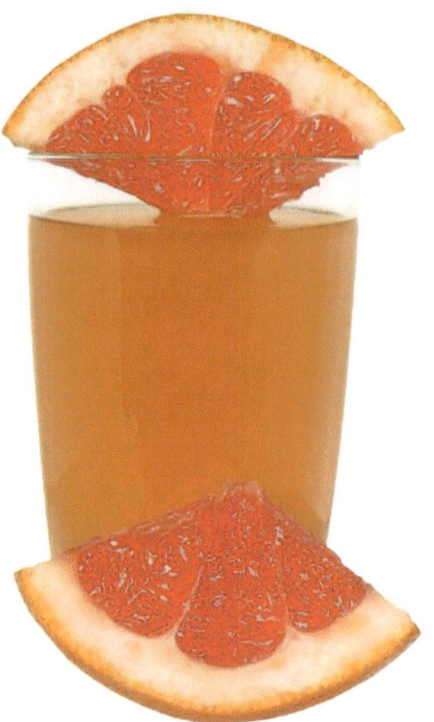

Preparation Time: 5 Min

Serves: 1

Ingredients:

- Grapefruit juice: 1 ½ cups.

- Apple cider vinegar: 1-2 tablespoons.

- Raw honey: 2 teaspoons.

Method

Mix all ingredients together and serve

Nutritional Information:

Contains iron, calcium, magnesium and manganese.

The Apple cider Shot

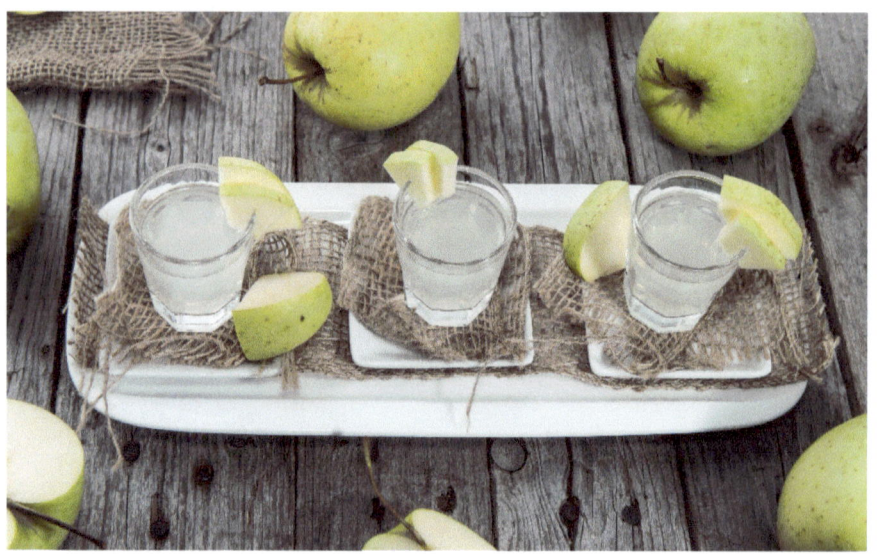

Preparation Time: 5 Min

Serves: 1

Ingredients:

- Apple cider vinegar: 1 tablespoon.

- Apple juice: 1 tablespoon

Method:

1. Mix all ingredients together and serve.

Nutritional Information:

Contains antioxidants.

Cider-Glazed Lamb Chops

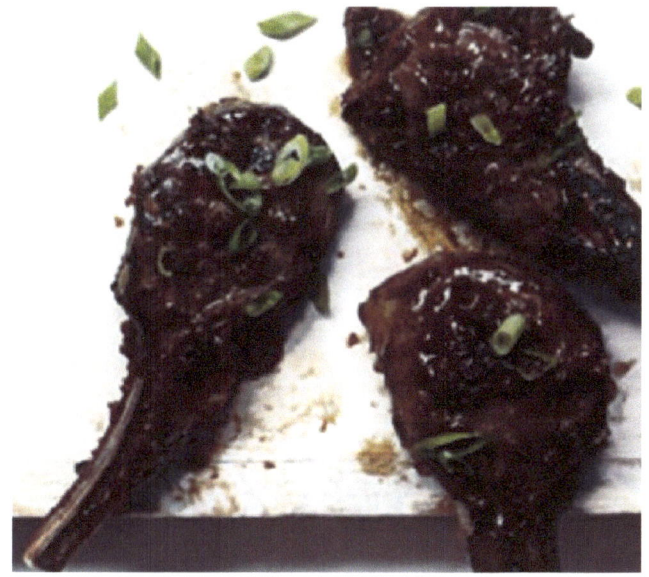

Preparation Time: 20 Min

Total Time: 40 Min

Serves: 4

Ingredients:

- Apple cider: 1 cup

- Minced and peeled ginger: 2 tablespoons

- Minced garlic: 2 tablespoons

- Soy sauce: 3 tablespoons

- Rice vinegar: 3 tablespoons

- Mild honey: 1 tablespoon

- Rib lamb chops, cut from 1 rack: 8

- Scallion, chopped: 1

Method:

1. Take a saucepan and boil the cider, soy sauce, garlic, honey and ginger for 12 minutes. When cool separate 2 tablespoons of the liquid to set aside.

2. Preheat your broiler.

3. Make sure lamb chops are dry. Season with salt. Brush the chops with the prepared glaze and broil them for 3 minutes each side.

4. Place on plate and pour over the reserved glaze.

5. Top with scallion.

Nutritional Information:

- Calories: 27

- Fat: 15 g

- Cholesterol: 102 mg

- Sodium: 866 mg

- Carbohydrates: 15g

- Fiber: 0.5 g

- Protein: 33 g

Classic apple chutney

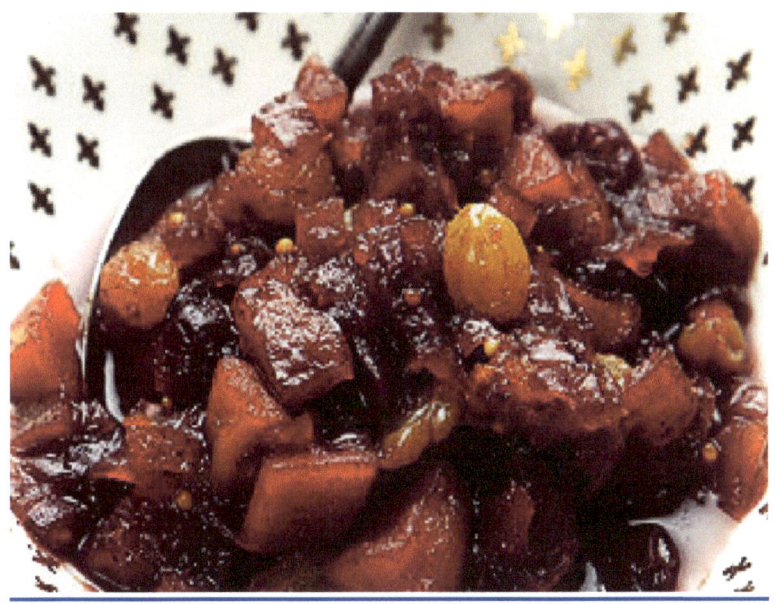

Preparation Time: 20-25 Min

Cooking Time: 40 Min

Total Time: 1 Hr. 10 Min

Ingredients:

- Apples peeled and diced: 1½ kg

- Light muscovado sugar: 750g

- Raisins: 500g

- Onion chopped: 2 medium

- Mustard seeds: 2 teaspoons

- Ground ginger: 2 teaspoons

- Salt: 1 teaspoon

- Cider vinegar: 700ml

Method:

1. Take a saucepan and boil the ingredients on a medium heat for 30-40 minutes.

2. When cool put into an air tight jar.

Nutritional Information:

- Calories: 123

- Fat: 1 g

- Carbohydrates: 32 g

- Fiber: 1 g

- Protein: 1 g

- Sugar: 19 g

- Salt: 0.17 g

Chapter 7: The Fun Stuff And Trivia About ACV

Did you know that...

… the Nobel Laureate (1912) in Medicine, Dr. Alexis Carrel from the Rockefeller Institute for Medical Research in New York kept chicken heart cells alive for 35 years – the life of a chicken is 7 years – with the help of ACV as a source of potassium?

… there are people who have lived up to 120 years – allegedly – owing to the daily use of ACV?

… that by adding 1 teaspoon of ACV to the water when cooking cauliflower keeps it looking white and appetizing?

… that if you add 1 tablespoon of ACV whilst cooking cabbage it eliminates unpleasant smells while boiling?

… you can quench your thirst quickly by drinking ACV mixed in cold water – 1 tablespoon per glass of water.

… applying a mix 1:1 ACV and water is a perfect treatment (and cure) for chapped skin? It heals quickly when treated with vinegar.

… you can make an excellent and fluffy meringue by beating3 egg whites and adding one teaspoon of ACV.

… peeled potatoes will not turn brown if you soak them in water and add 2-3 drops of ACV? The potatoes can be stored like this in the refrigerator for about 10 days.

… you can store pimentos and olives forever if they are submerged in ACV?

… you can pickle ANYTHING in ACV? It is a universal pickling agent.

… about 10 per cent of all the vinegar produced in the USA goes for the making of ketchup and mayonnaise?

… the ACV's boiling point is 213 degrees Fahrenheit?

… vinegar was part and parcel of the military for a very long time in history? It was kept in all army hospitals as a highly effective, low-cost disinfectant. It was also used to keep the guns and cannons unfrozen and rust-free. This goes back to Medieval times.

… ACV is so potent in killing bacteria, viruses and other harmful agents that it can immunize against even plague? In the 1300s, people condemned (to death) were "hired" to help clean the dead bodies of people who died of the plague. Four of those survived. It was later found out that they drank copious amounts of vinegar with pickled garlic in it.

… not all glass is safe to store ACV (and any vinegar) in? There is lead glass; if you store vinegar in a lead glass, it will become poison.

… soaking your freshly painted nails in a ½ cup of warm water in which 2 tablespoons of ACV is mixed will ensure that your nail polish will stay put for a much longer time?

… you can make acne disappear in days by applying ACV directly to the spots with the help of Q-tips?

… you can easily remove a splinter wedged in the body by soaking the part of the body in ACV for about 20 minutes? The splinter becomes loose, and you can remove it easily.

…you can eliminate litter pan odor by wiping with 1:1 solution of water and vinegar? It also kills the bacteria.

Conclusion: ACV In Your Life

When you are reading this last part of the Book, you will have realized the huge potential this simple compound has to change your life around for the better. It is not much to ask, drinking a few glasses every day and watching your diet.

The returns are so unimaginably rich. You get to be healthy, you get to fight cancer, you get to live a very long time, and you tend to be able to conquer dementia and Alzheimer's disease – and so much more. No more creaking bones, no more arthritis, no more mucus choking you from inside out, no more yeast infections, no more fungal infections and so on.

Apple Cider Vinegar can bring plenty of joy to your life. Whether you are drinking it as a tonic, use it on salads or as a cleaner, ACV has something to provide for everybody. Research agrees to most of the claims of the health benefits of ACV.

It is sad and even tragic that people worldwide are still ill informed about this amazing compound. Hopefully, books such as this will act as eye-openers that urge people to return to the gifts of Mother Nature, who has a solution for everything.

I sincerely hope you enjoyed reading this Book, just as I much enjoyed putting it together.

Have fun and stay healthy!

Cheers!

Helpful Resources

Free eBooks About ACV

1. ACV for Cleaning - http://www.health-womens-healthy-living-goals.com/support-files/vinegar-for-cleaning.pdf

2. ACV for Health - http://www.health-womens-healthy-living-goals.com/support-files/vinegar-for-health.pdf

3. Lather Lass eBook – All About Apple Cider Vinegar - http://latherlass.com/wp-content/uploads/LatherLass-eBook-v1.3.pdf

4. Herb Wisdom – Apple Cider Vinegar - http://www.herbwisdom.com/herb-apple-cider-vinegar.html

5. 20 Pain Cures from Your Kitchen - http://www.iitk.ac.in/hc/20_Pain_Cures_in_Our_Kitchen_Cupboard.pdf

Helpful Sites and Articles

1. Recommendation of ACV by Simon Yu, MD, Board Certified Internist, who practices medicine with focus on Alternative Medicine -

http://www.preventionandhealing.com/articles/Apple_Cider_Vinegar.pdf

2. Apple Cider Vinegar for your Dog -
    http://essentiallydogs.com/apple-cider-vinegar-for-dogs

3. Cleaning Recipes Using Vinegar -
    http://www.goodgirlgonegreen.com/7-diy-cleaning-recipes-using-vinegar/

4. How to ACV for Beautiful Hair and Skin -
    http://www.huffingtonpost.com/organic-authoritycom/apple-cider-vinegar-beauty_b_1924171.html?ir=India&adsSiteOverride=in

5. All About Apple Cider Vinegar -
    http://cider.org.uk/frameset.htm

6. 101 Uses of Apple Cider Vinegar -
    http://andreadekker.com/101-more-uses-for-vinegar/

7. Home Remedies with Apple Cider Vinegar -
    http://homeremedieslog.com/natural-products/foods/apple-cider-vinegar/

Recipes with ACV

1. How to Make Apple Cider Vinegar at Home - http://cookforgood.com/recipe/homemade-organic-apple-cider-vinegar.html

2. Recipes of ACV Drinks - http://onehundredoneways2life.hubpages.com/hub/Apple-Cider-Vinegar-Recipes

3. Recipes with ACV - http://www.countryliving.com/food-drinks/g1028/cider-recipes/?slide=1

4. ACV Drink Tonic Recipe - http://thehealthyeatingsite.com/apple-cider-vinegar-drink-recipe-basic-tonic/

5. Salad Vinaigrette - http://www.food.com/recipe/apple-cider-vinegar-and-honey-vinaigrette-dressing-396343

6. ACV Detox Drinks - http://www.healthyandnaturalworld.com/apple-cider-vinegar-detox-drinks/

7. Recipes that use ACV - http://www.thekitchn.com/from-doughnuts-to-sorbet-10-recipes-that-use-apple-cider-179242

Polite note, if you found this eBook helpful in any way kindly post a review.

Check out more books by Global Heaven Publishing

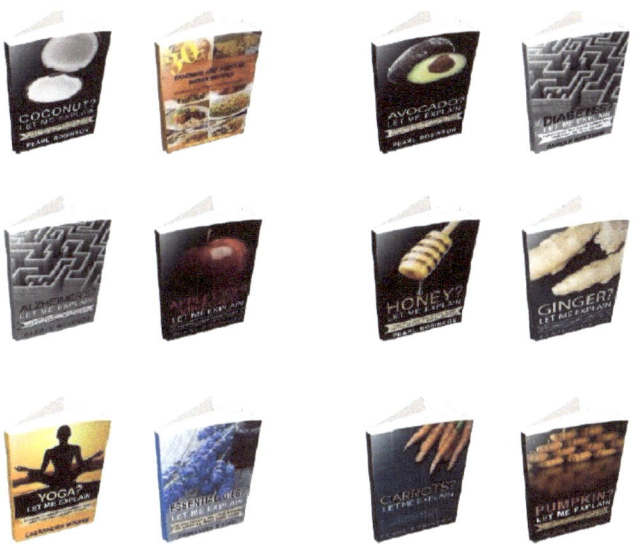

www.ingramcontent.com/pod-product-compliance
Lightning Source LLC
Chambersburg PA
CBHW040310010626
45792CB00022B/30